PATCH LAND ADVENTURES

BOOK TWO

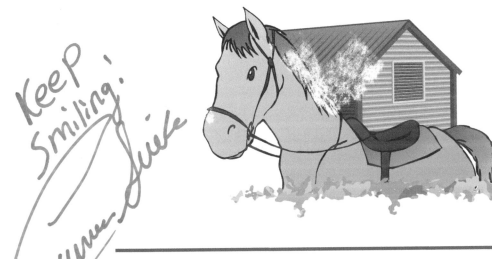

Keep Smiling!

CAMPING AT MIMI'S RANCH

WRITTEN BY CARMEN SWICK
ILLUSTRATED BY JOEY MANFRE

For information go to: www.presbeaupublishing.com or email carmens222@gmail.com

The author of this book does not dispense medical advice or prescribe the use of any technique as a form of treatment physical or emotional, or medical problems without the advice of a physician, either directly or indirectly. The intent of the author is to share her story about her son and to help those with eye patching to be able to use this book as a tool, and for the children that do not need to eye patch, they will enjoy the fiction adventures the story delivers.

Carmen Swick's Editor: Page Lambert

Illustrator: Joey Manfre

Cover design by: Joey Manfre

Carmen Swick's Head Shot by: MDphotonet.com

PRESBEAU PUBLISHING

Publisher: Presbeau Publishing Inc.

ISBN# 978-0-9831380-4-4

Second Edition

Library of Congress Control Number: 2015914260

Printed and Bound and Published in the United States of America

Patch Land Adventures: Camping at Mimi's Ranch www.patchlandadventures.com

FOREWARD

Carmen Swick's books will hopefully help children to accept their own patches or encourage support of one another to patch faithfully when necessary, thus helping to improve amblyopia outcomes. I applaud Ms. Swick's efforts to this end and congratulate her son Preston for being an inspiration to his mother and to children who are faced with amblyopia themselves or in a friend or family member.

Dr. Diana DeSantis, MD.

I admire the author for following her heart in creating awareness about amblyopia. Carmen's Patch Land Adventures series helps parents as well as children cope with the diagnosis of amblyopia. While children are afraid that the patch will limit their ability to carry on with normal activities and their social interactions with peers, parents are struck with the challenge of how to handle their children s `emotional turbulence as they enforce a new regimen. In this book, Carmen has found a way to ease the difficulties of patching with a delightful story that demonstrates patching can be easy. Children will feel at ease immediately when they see that they can still fish, walk the dog, play ball, etc.

Dr. Elizabeth K. Thomas, O.D.

Patch Land Adventures 2: Camping at Mimi's Ranch is a warmhearted tale that will captivate and delight children of all ages. Swick has a talent for weaving education, inspiration and joy into one powerful little story. Preston and his friends are infectious their experiences and adventures are both amusing and relatable The Patch Land Adventures series is a perfect collection for parents, teachers, doctors, children or anyone.

Melissa Kline, Author of *My Beginning* and *Storm*

A creative tool to help children who are living with a medical or physical challenge overcome fears and build confidence. This heart-warming story will also help children understand the unique differences among people from all walks of life.

Kristin Miller, Editor-in-Chief, *Denver Life Magazine*

PATCH LAND ADVENTURES

EXTRAS!

After reading the story, please continue on to our Bonus Pages!

Includes:

A Study Guide

Information Chart

2 Coloring Pages

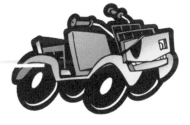

DEDICATIONS AND ACKNOWLEDGMENTS

This book is dedicated to my son Preston who truly inspired me to write Patch Land Adventures book and turn it into a series. Patching did not stop Preston from doing what he loves! Preston's diligence in patching to help improve his eyesight was outstanding. He was committed to the efforts required and pushed ahead through the tough times and set-backs. I love you and thank you for not giving up.

Special thanks, to my family and friends for their support and believing I could write our story to share with many. Mimi thank you for always being so supportive and creative with all the incentive packages you sent Preston to stay on course.

Page Lambert, my editor, you were so kind and patient with me and not only helped with the editing, you also guided me through the process.

Joey Manfre, my illustrator, thank you for bringing Book Two: "Camping at Mimi's Ranch" to life with your illustrations and being my my creative partner, to help tell the story through the author's vision! Your gift as an artist truly shows through your work. I am happy to say that I have also found a friend.

Let's not forget our dog Beau who is a Weimaraner, Preston's eye patch buddy in the Patch Land Adventures. Beau has a very special bond with Preston.

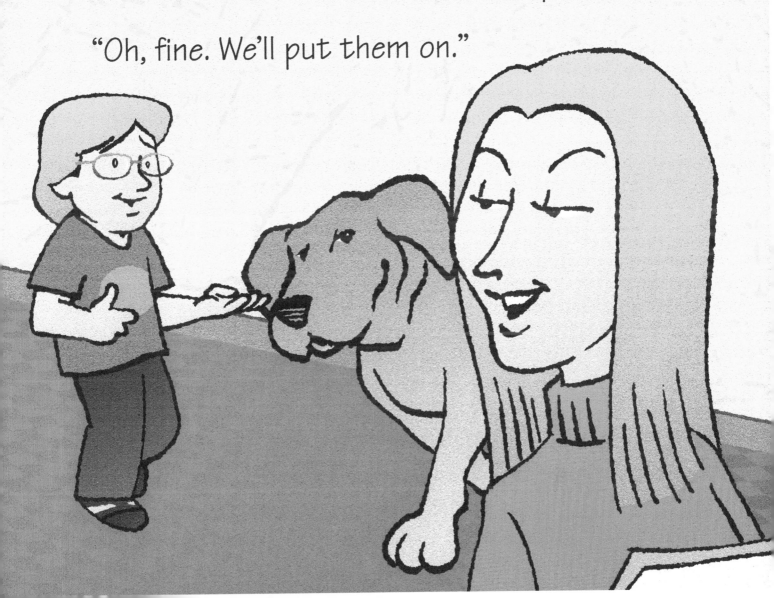

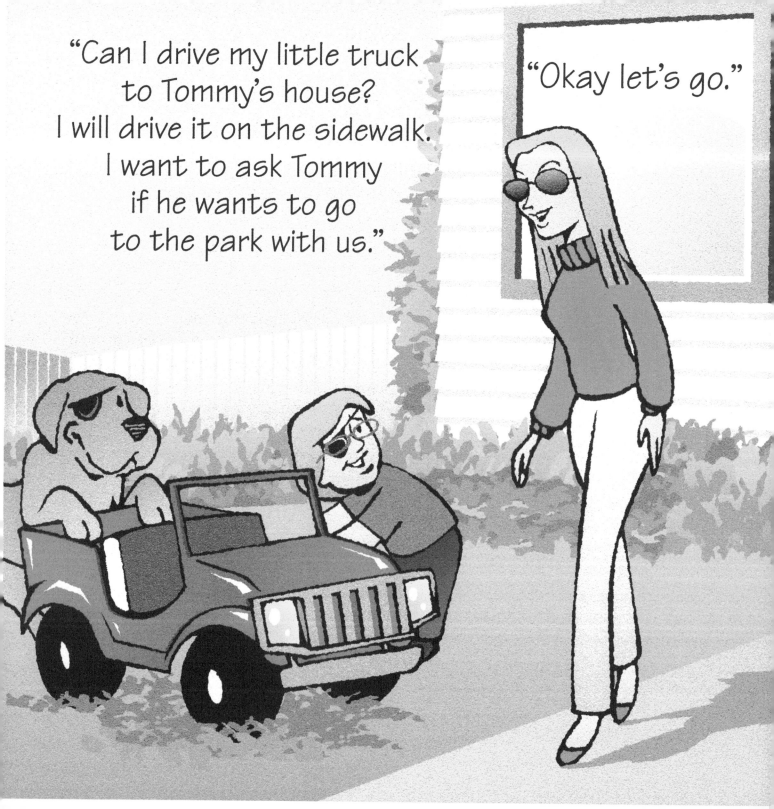

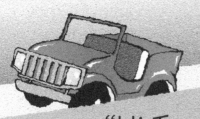

"Hi Tommy. Can you go to the park?"

"My mom said 'yes' if I put my eye patch on."

"Put it on. We can do anything with an eye patch on."

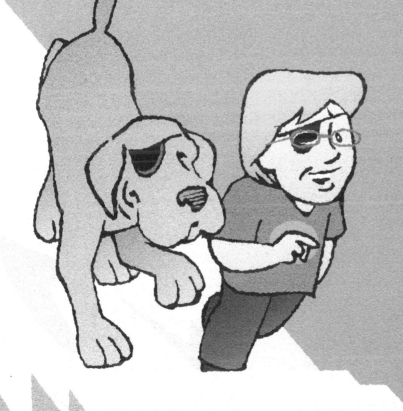

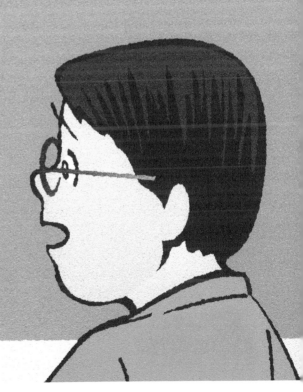

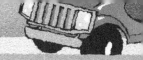

"Guess what? At night, I get to go to Patch Land. If you want to go, all you have to do before you go to sleep is put your eye patch under your pillow."

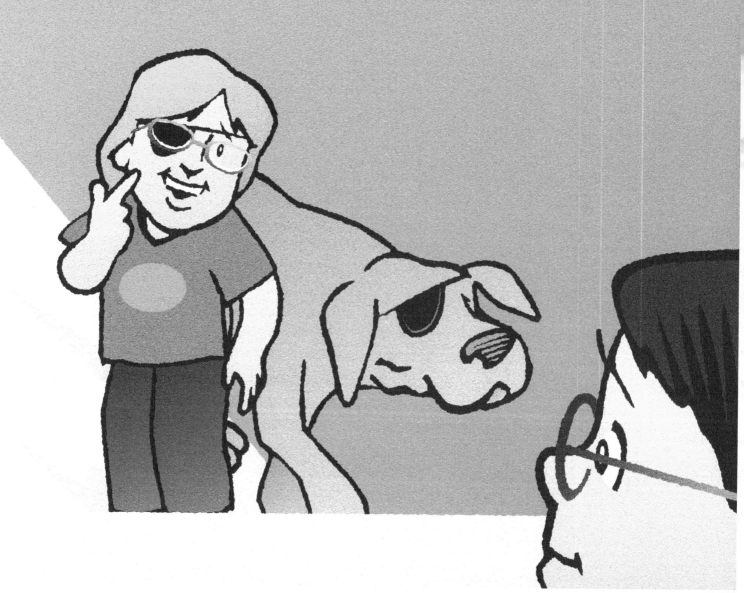

"There are other kids and animals there. Everyone wears an eye patch. You can always see Beau and me there. Beau is always there because he is my patch buddy and he goes everywhere with me. It is lots of fun."

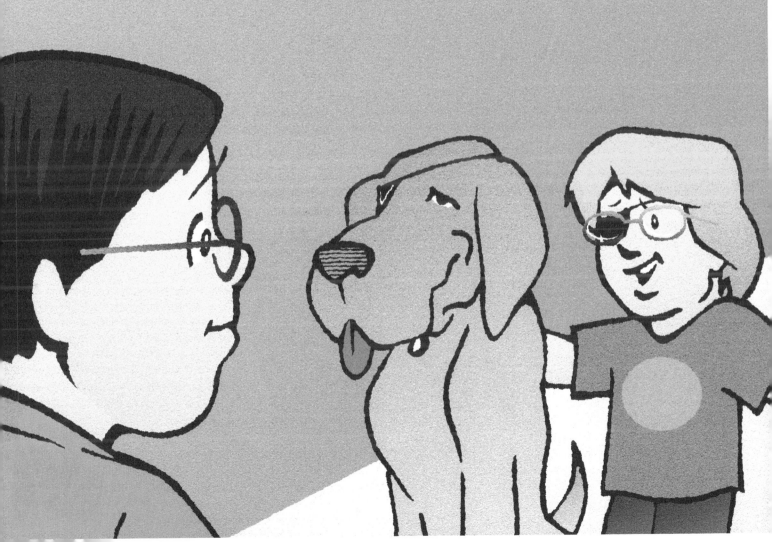

"Preston, I just don't like my patch. It's not cool."

"Tommy, my mom and dad bought me some cool ones. I got to pick them out. Ask your mom and dad to buy you some cool ones. Now put your patch on and let's go to the park!"

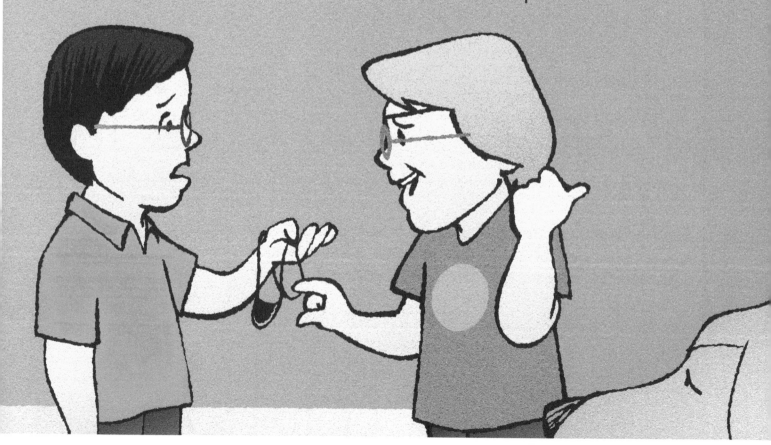

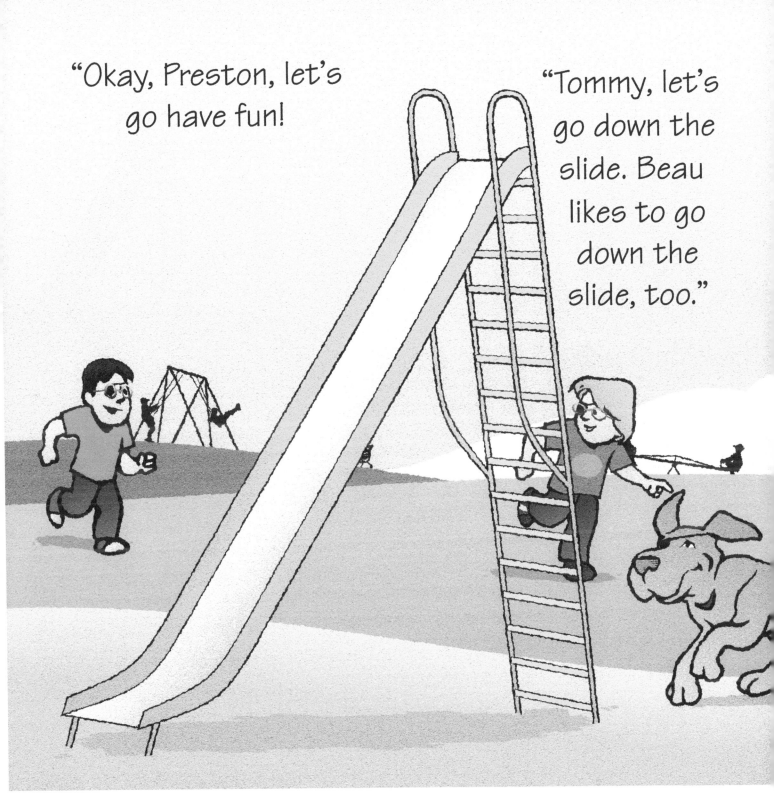

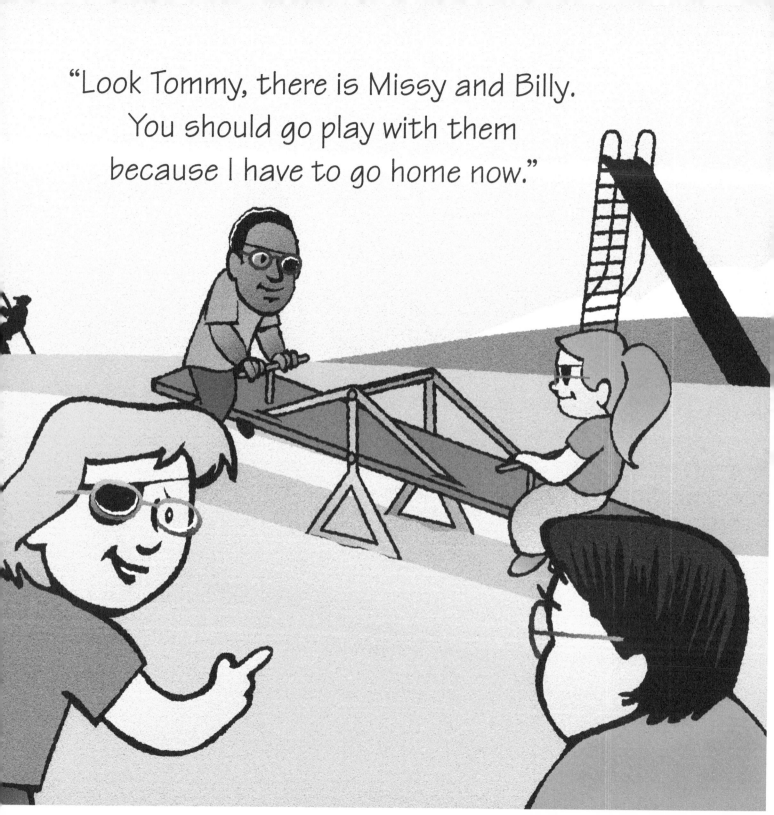

"Why do you have to leave?"

"Mom says we are going camping at Mimi's ranch. I will get to ride my favorite horse, Winston."

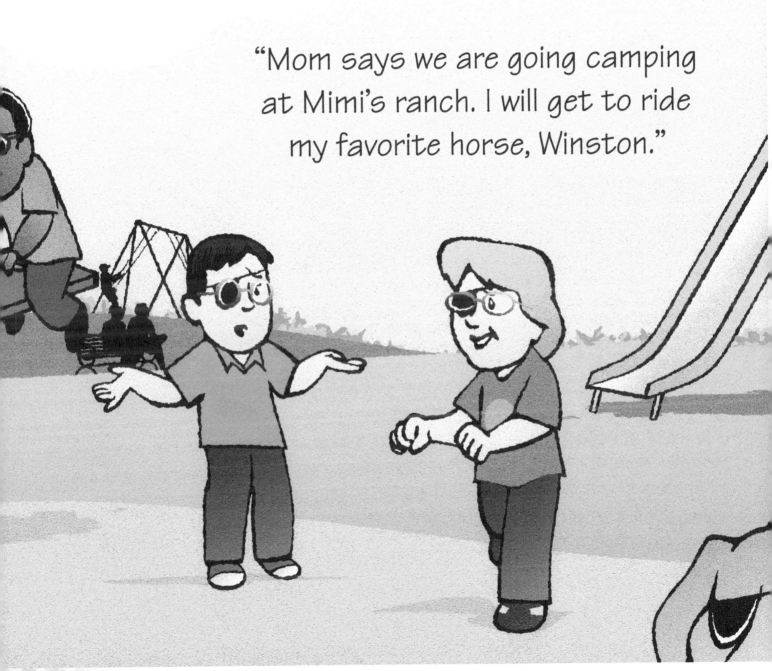

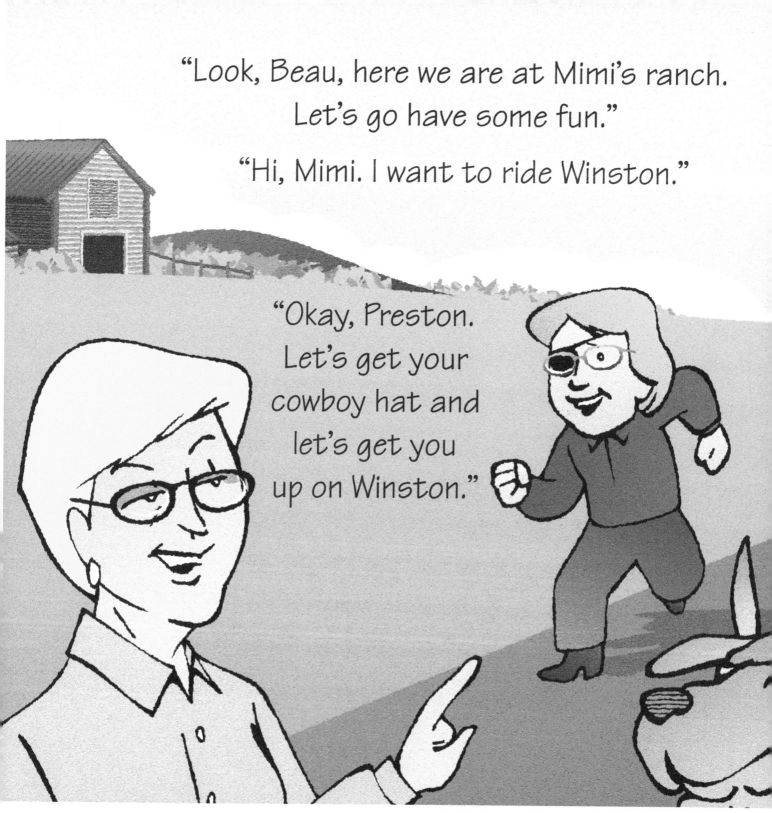

"Beau, come on and follow Mimi and me.
Mimi is going to lead Winston with a lead rope."

"Giddy up, giddy up, horsy!
I can ride a horse with my eye patch on.
We can do anything!"

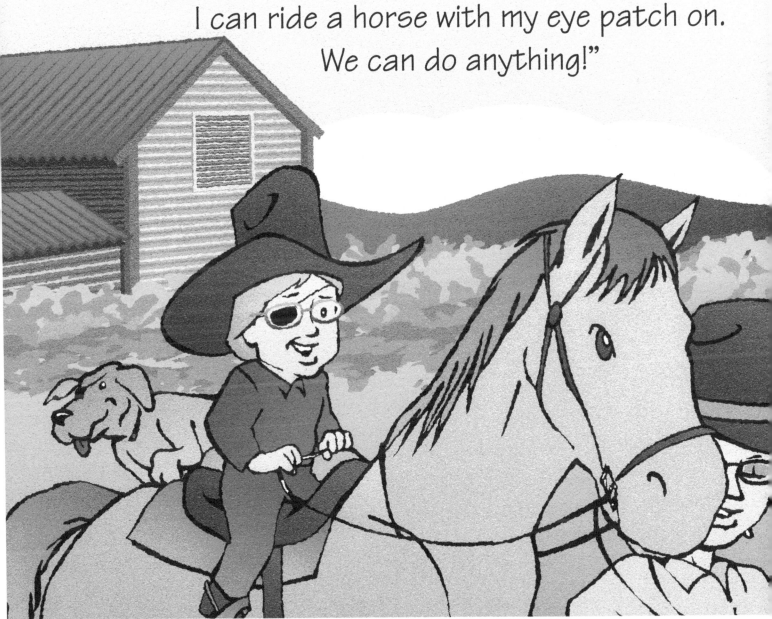

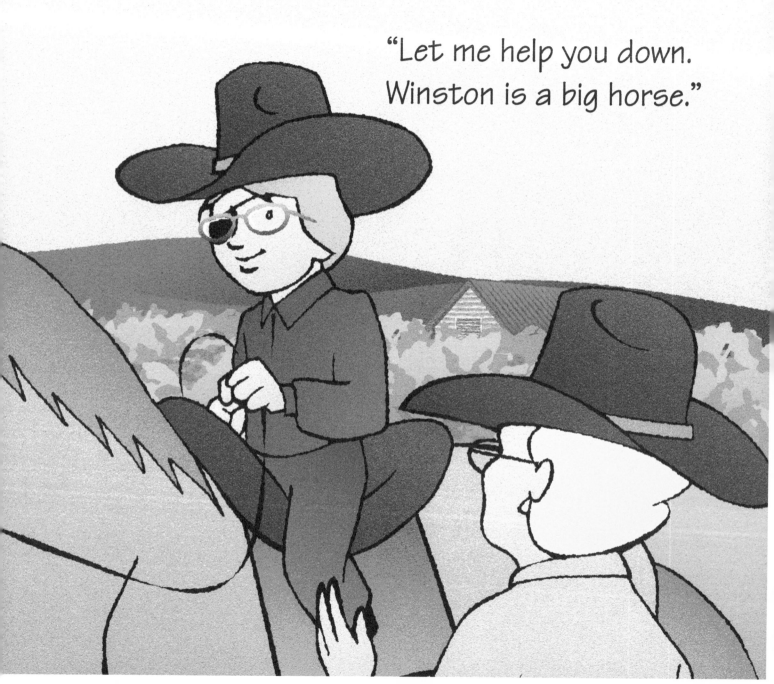

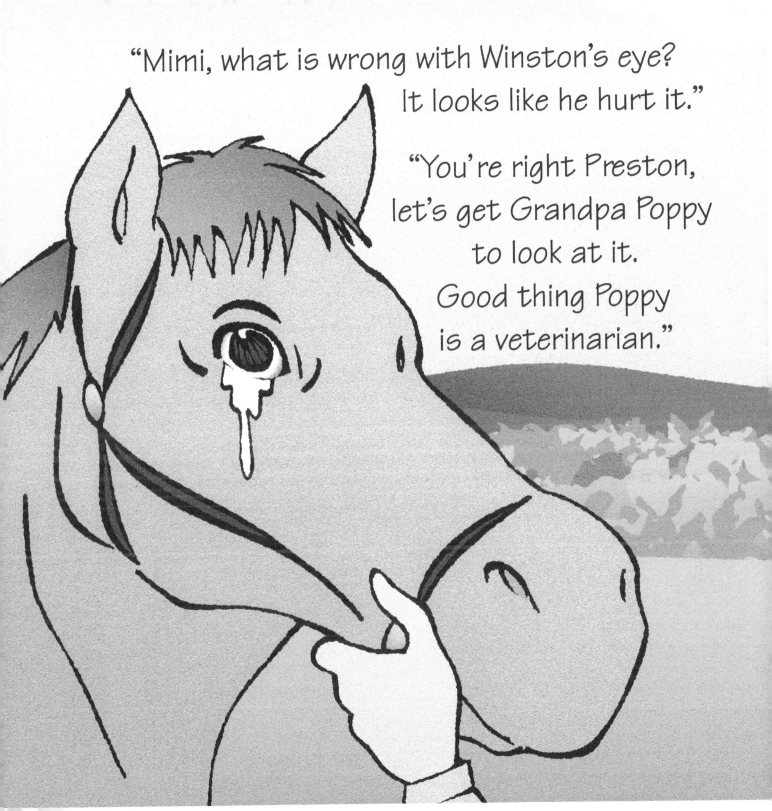

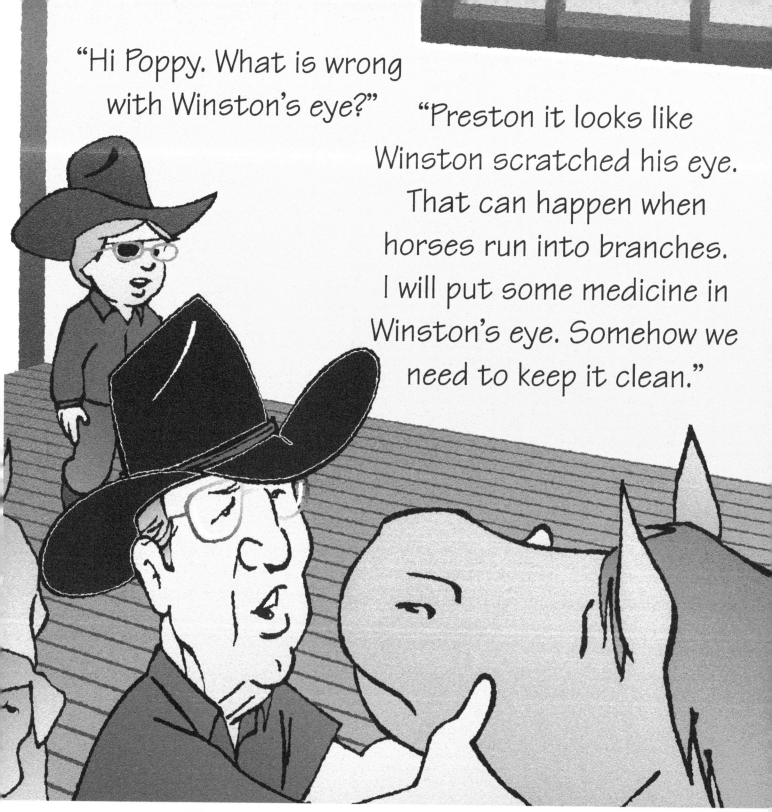

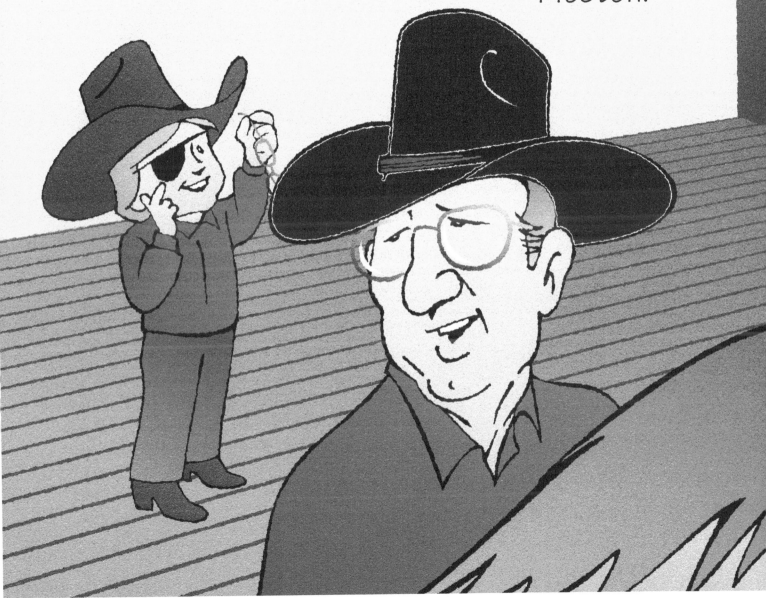

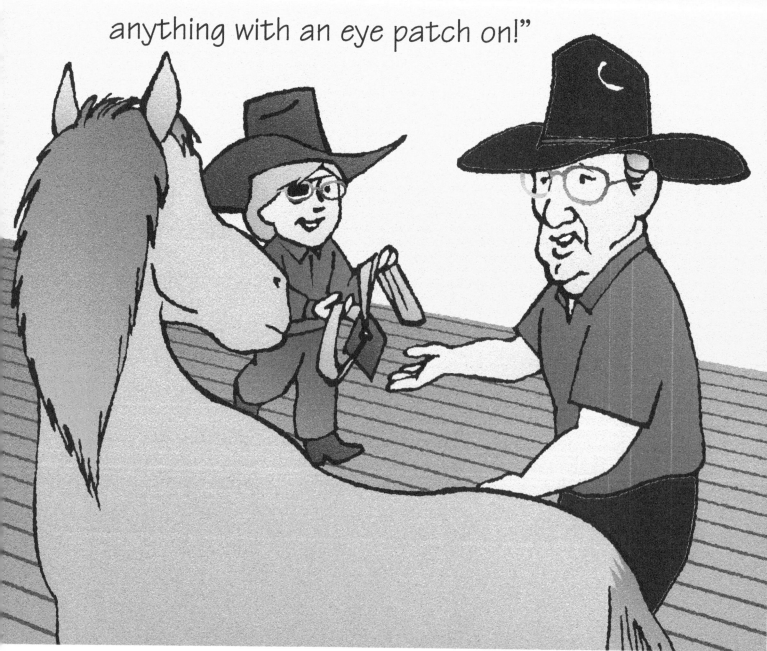

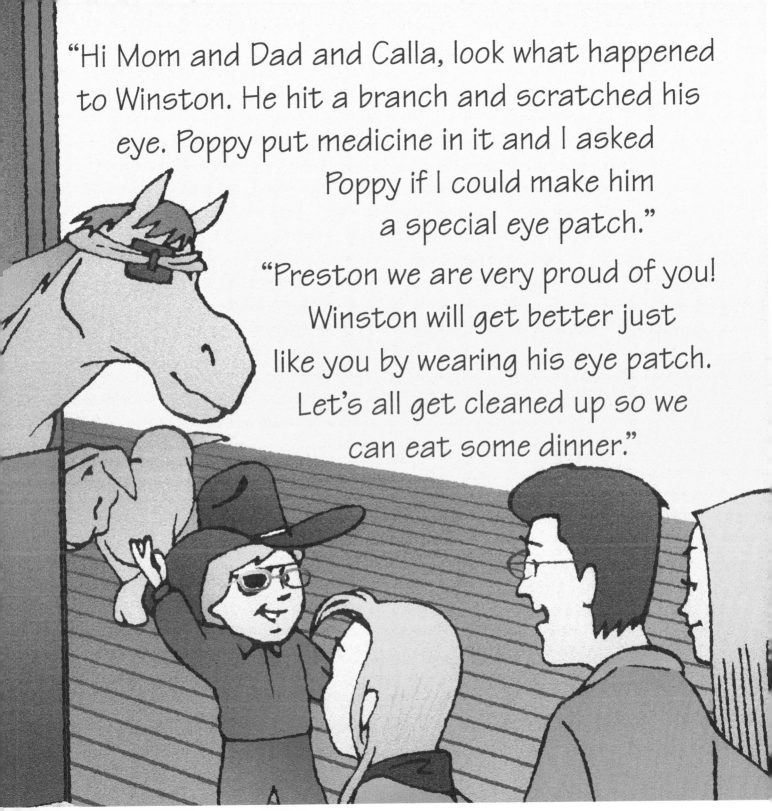

"Hi Mom and Dad and Calla, look what happened to Winston. He hit a branch and scratched his eye. Poppy put medicine in it and I asked Poppy if I could make him a special eye patch."

"Preston we are very proud of you! Winston will get better just like you by wearing his eye patch. Let's all get cleaned up so we can eat some dinner."

"It is getting late. We need to get you ready for bed."

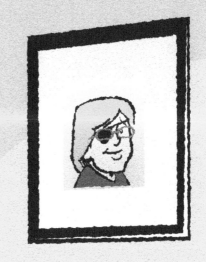

"Okay, Mimi. I can't wait to go to Patch Land!"

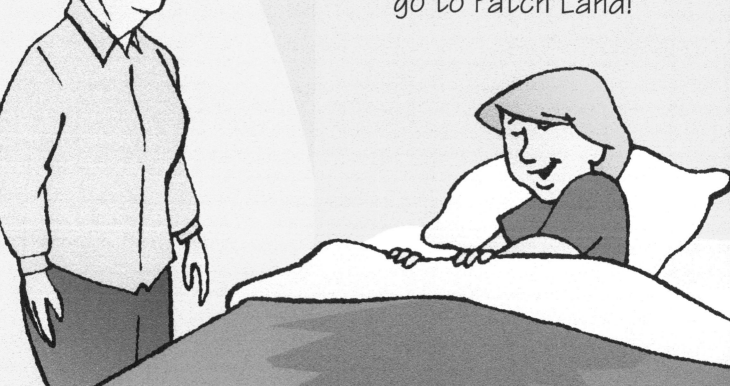

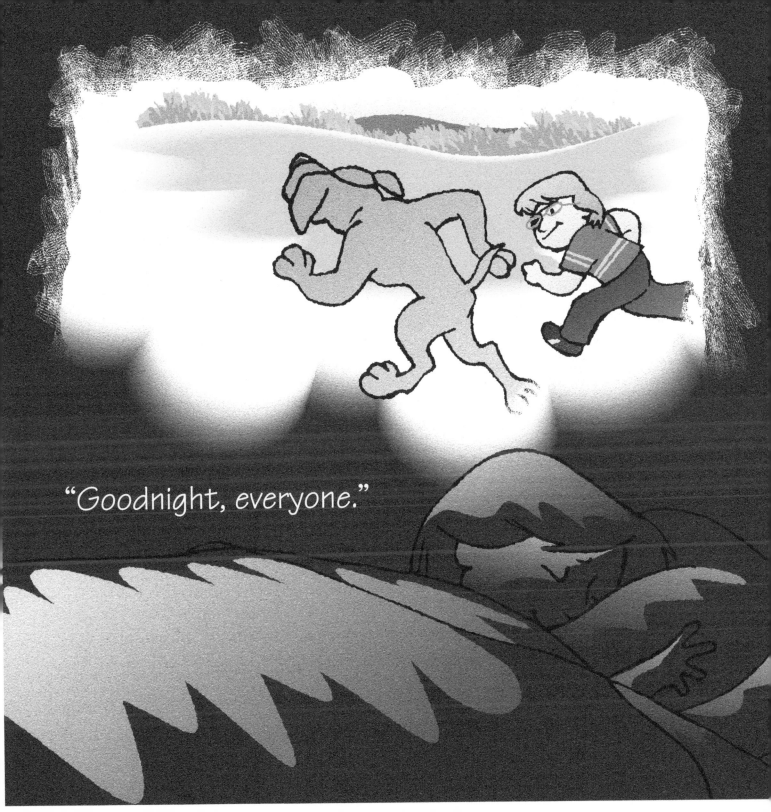

"Goodnight, everyone."

"Beau, here we are in Patch Land. Tommy and Winston might be here tonight. I see Winston. Look, there's Tommy. I told you it was easy to come to Patch Land."

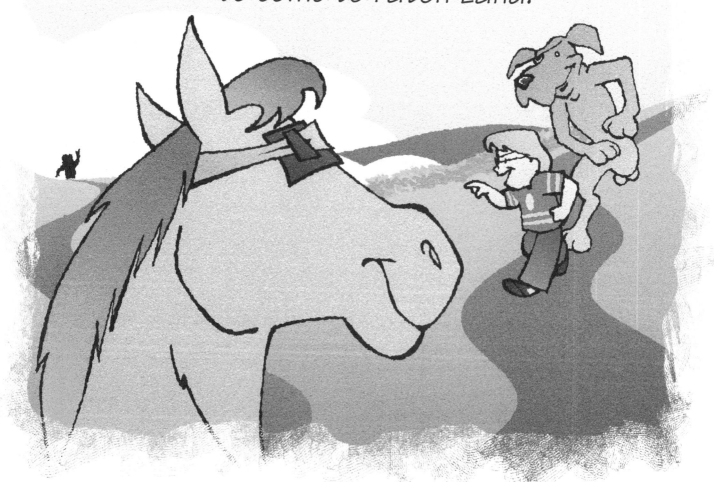

"Preston, is that Winston?
What happened to his eye?"

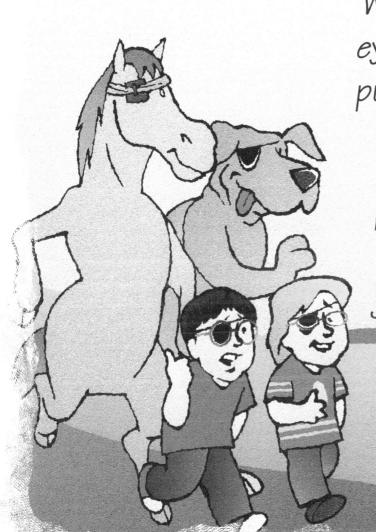

"Winston scratched his
eye on a branch. Poppy
put medicine in his eye,
and I made him his
special eye patch.
He has to wear it till
his eye gets better.
Just like we have to."

"Tommy, put your helmet on and get on your 4-wheeler. You and Winston follow Beau and me."
"I want to show you both all the animals here and their cool eye patches. Now, let's go have some fun."

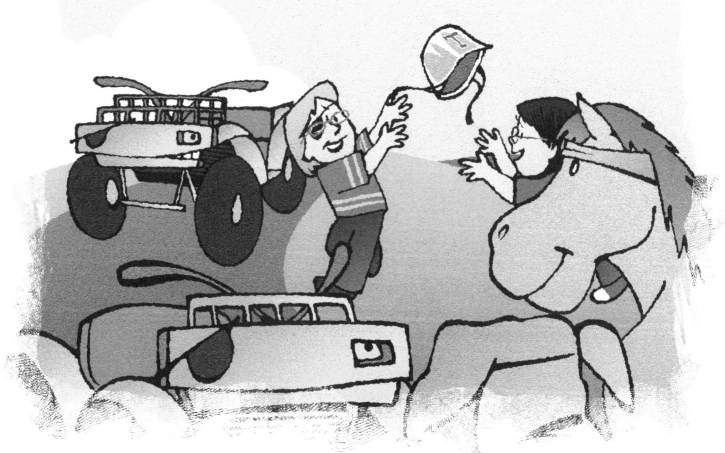

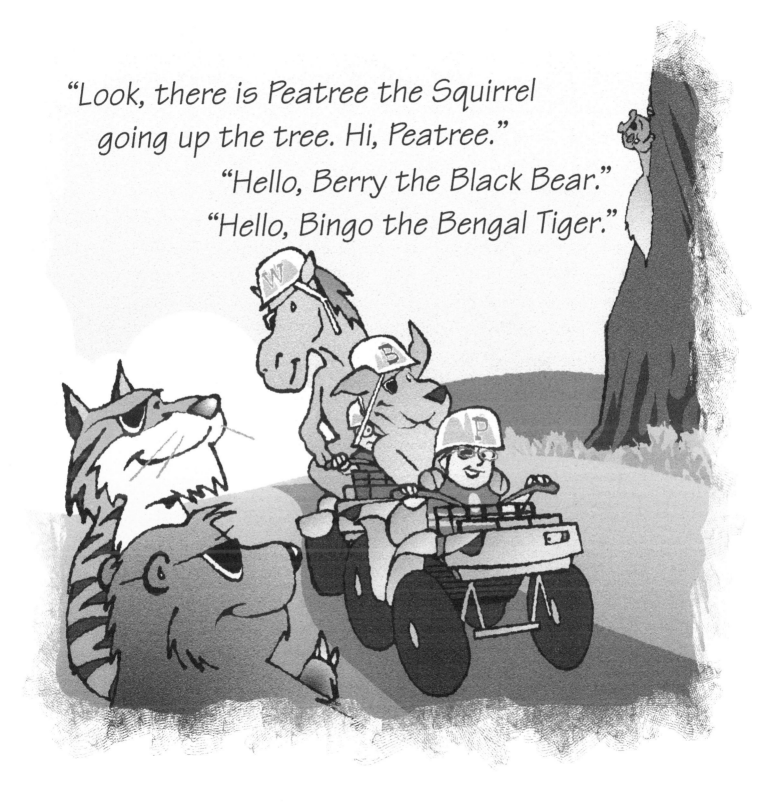

"Look, Tommy, there is Pout the Brook Trout.
Jumping high in the sky. Out of the brook!
Back in the brook!"

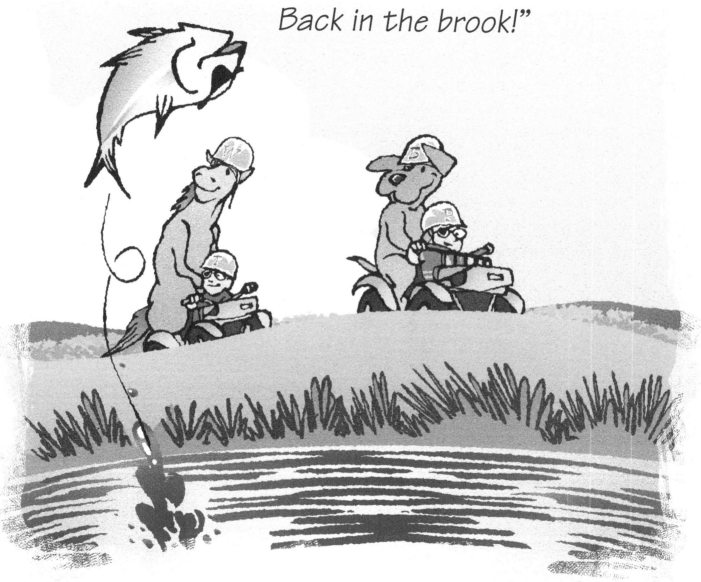

"Stinky the Skunk is by the stump. Slinky the Snake and Foxy the Fox and Snort the Pig are there too. Isn't this fun, Tommy?"

"Yes, it is! Let's go see more animals."

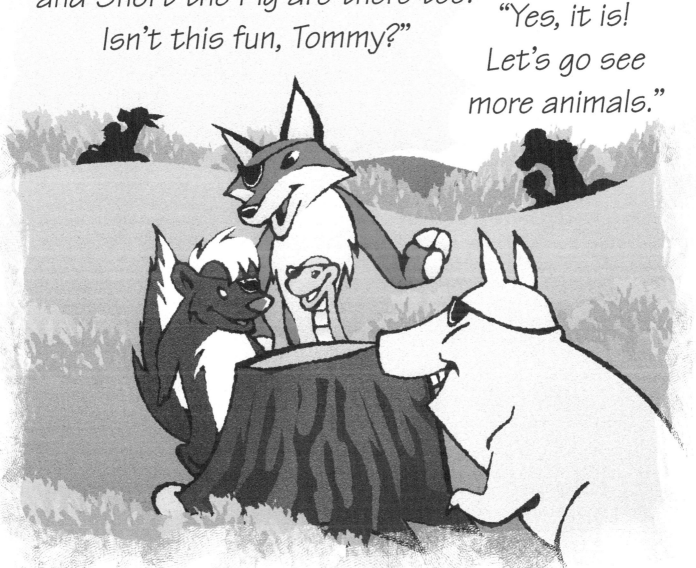

"Sorry, Tommy we need to go. Mimi is trying to wake me up but you can go have fun until your mom wakes you up."

"Okay. Bye Preston. Thank you for telling me about Patch Land."

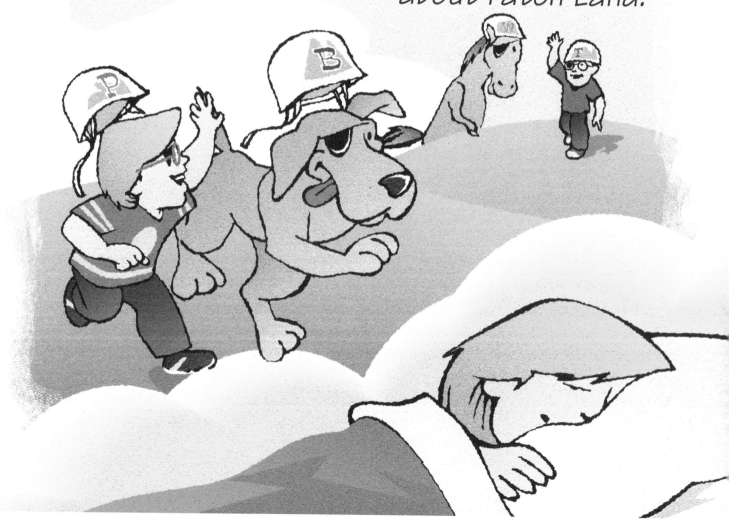

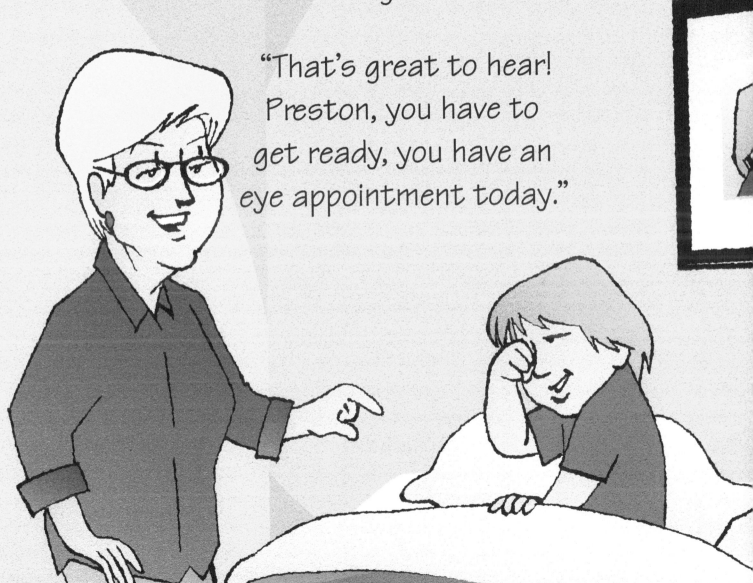

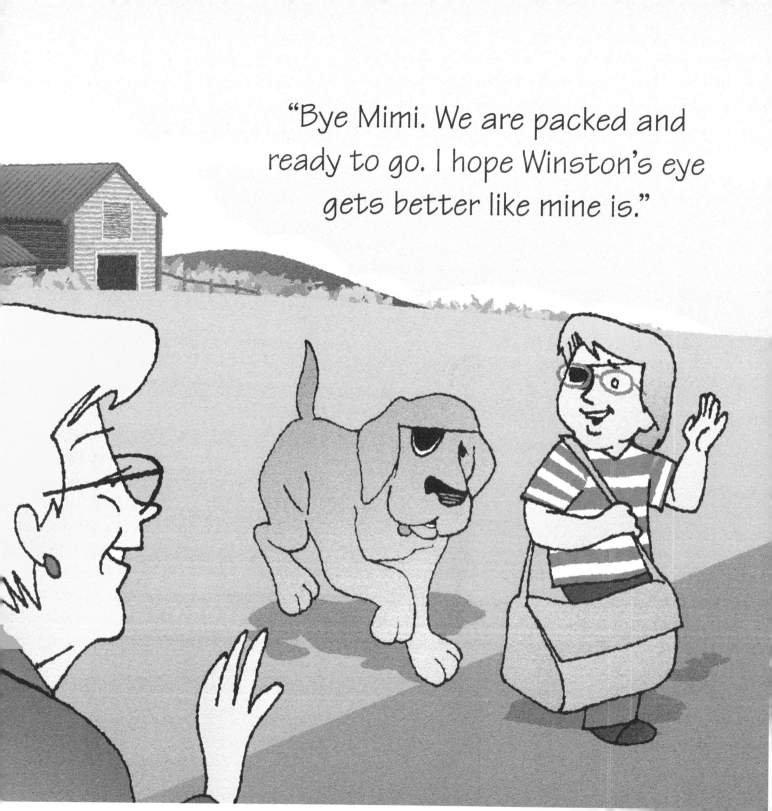

"Bye Mimi. We are packed and ready to go. I hope Winston's eye gets better like mine is."

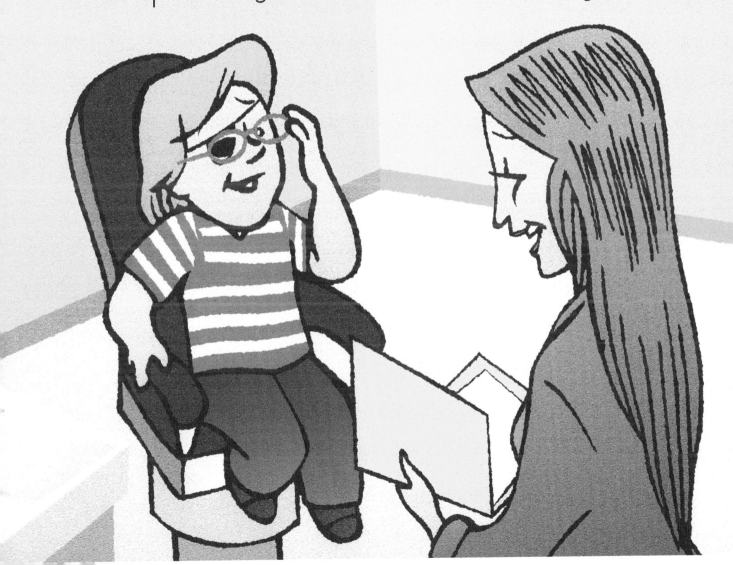

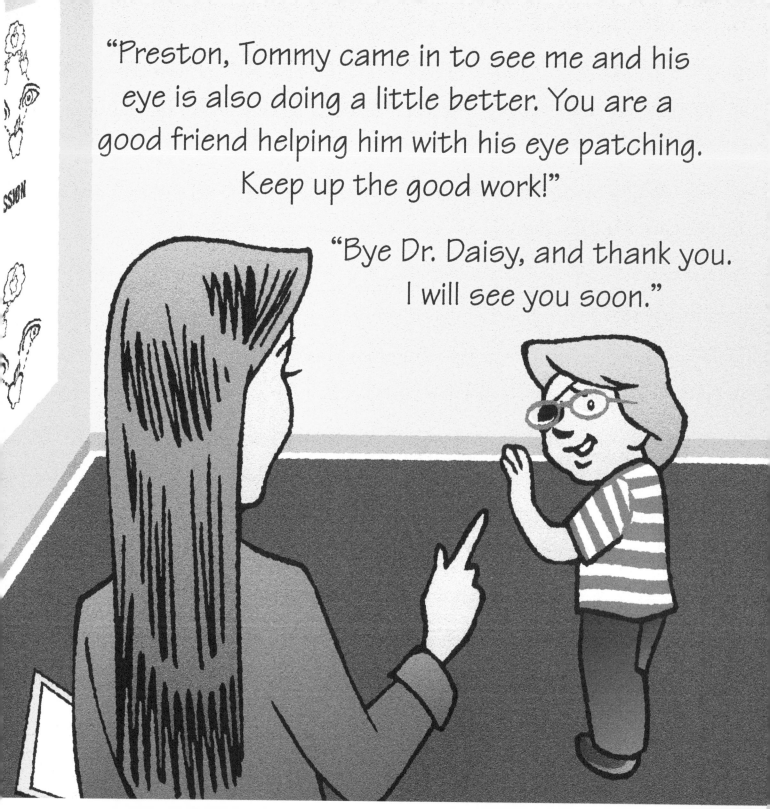

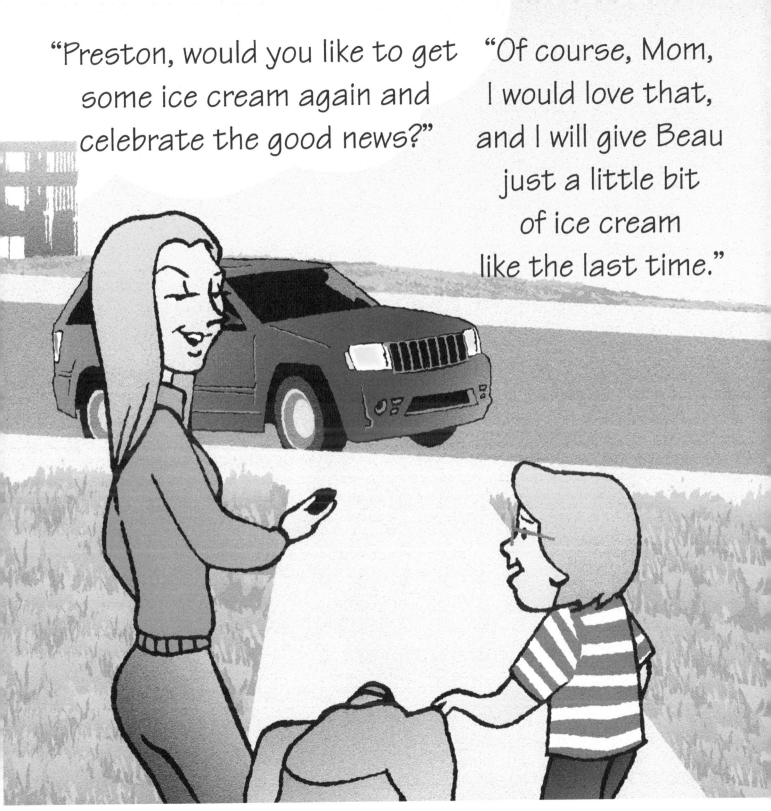

"Mom, it was so much fun in Patch Land last night. Tommy and Winston were there with Beau and me. Can't wait to go back again and I hope they go too."

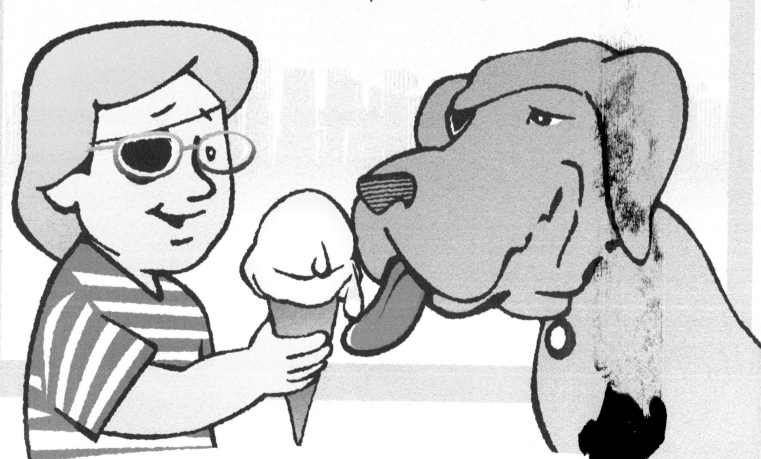

PATCH LAND ADVENTURES

BOOK TWO
WORK SHEET/COMPREHENSION

Name:

Date:

1) Why does Preston have to wear an eye patch?

2) What is the name of Preston's dog?

3) Who's ranch does Preston go to?

4) What is the horse's name?

5) Preston has a friend that he helps with his eye patching. What is his friend's name?

6) How does Preston go to Patch Land at night?

7) Can you name a few of the animals in Patch Land?

8) What is the name of Preston's eye doctor?

9) What is the author's name?

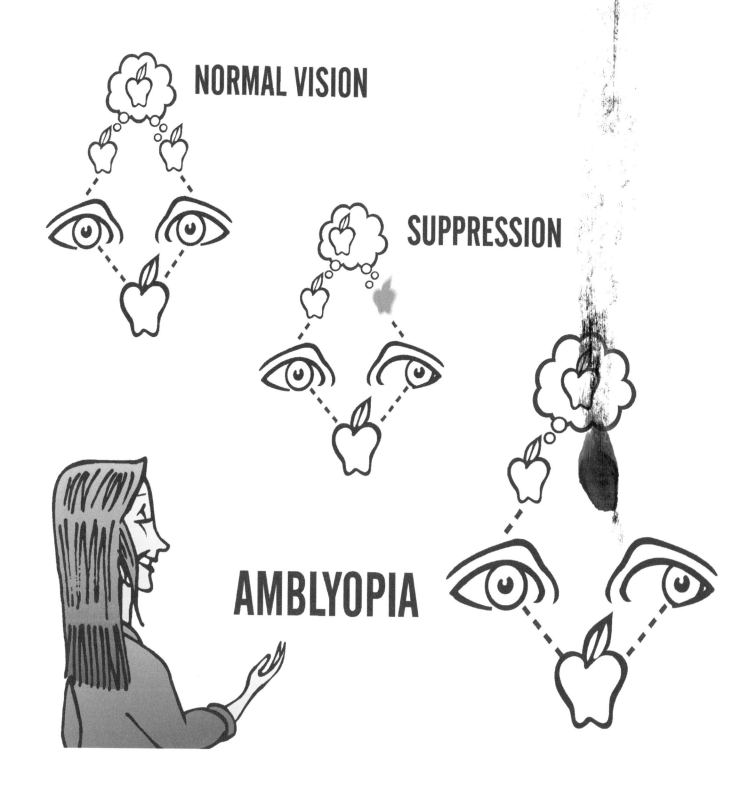

ABOUT AMBLYOPIA

Amblyopia is the leading cause of blindness in children. A condition in which a person's vision does not develop properly in early childhood because the eye and the brain are not working together correctly. Amblyopia, which usually affects only one eye, is also known as "lazy eye." A person with amblyopia experiences blurred vision in the affected eye. However, children often do not complain of blurred vision in the amblyopic eye because this seems normal to them. Early treatment is advisable, because if left untreated, this condition may lead to permanent vision problems.

For more information visit: Prevent Blindness at: http://www.preventblindness.org

Also Children's Eye Foundation: http://www.childrenseyefoundation.org

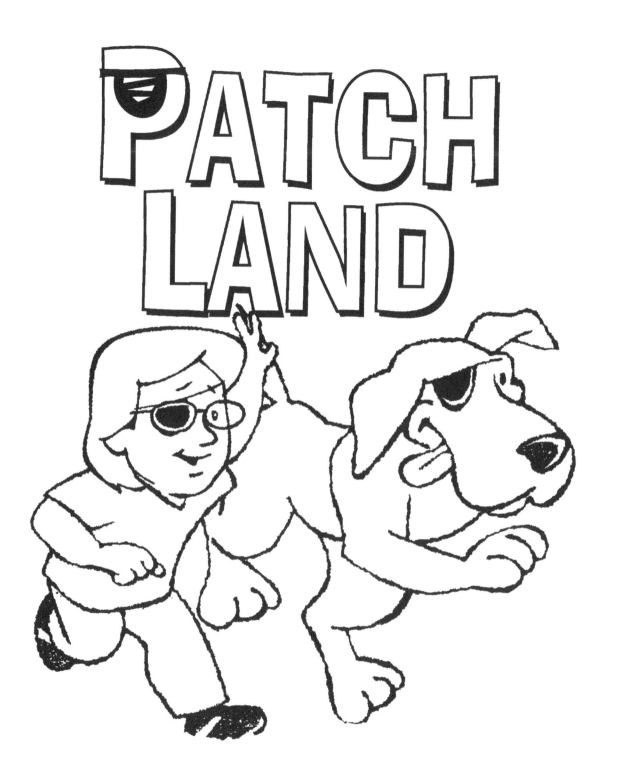

PATCH LAND

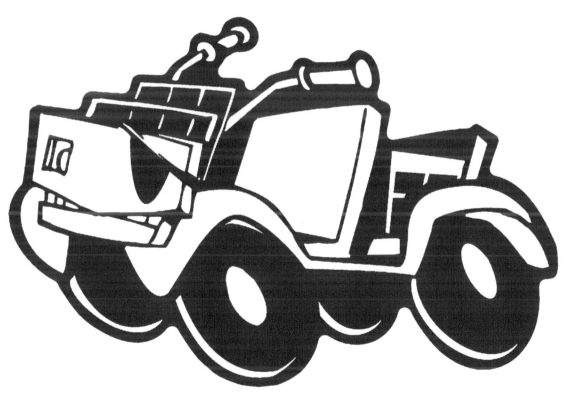

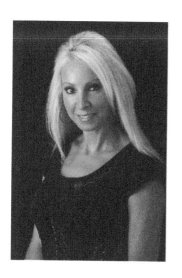

ABOUT THE AUTHOR

Author and speaker Carmen Swick lives in Colorado with her family where they enjoy many of the outdoor activities that the Centennial State has to offer. She volunteers with a non-profit organization, The Foundation Fighting Blindness, where she holds the position as President of the Denver Chapter. Outside of The Foundation Fighting Blindness she is the Chair for The Blind Taste of the Rockies, which is an annual fundraiser to raise awareness and search for a cure to blindness. In 2012 Carmen led the role of Chair for the Denver Vision Walk all the while attending schools for presentations/workshops and signings for the Patch Land Adventure series. Helping to find a cure for blindness isn't her only passion; she leads a team in the role of Captain in the Race for the Cure. She was the presenting children's book author for the 2014 Young Writers Conference for Jeffco Elementary Schools.

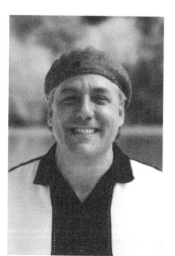

ABOUT THE ILLUSTRATOR

Joey Manfre is an illustrator and graphic artist with over twenty years of professional experience. Based in Northern California, he has worked on projects ranging from fancy wine packaging to funky tee shirts, but has a special fondness for illustrating books. For more information, check out his online portfolio at www.behance.net/joeyofdrawing.

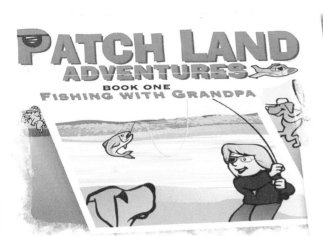
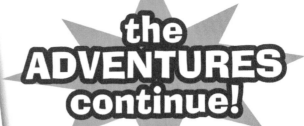
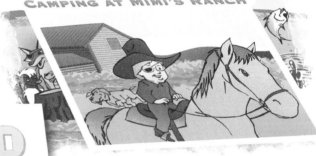
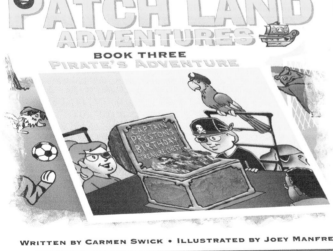
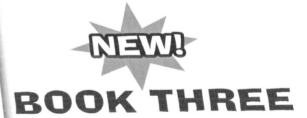

CPSIA information can be obtained
at www.ICGtesting.com
Printed in the USA
FSOW03n0124011015
11714FS

9 780983 138044